Generalized Anxiety Disorder

The Most Practical Guide on How to Be Calmer, Learn to Defeat Anger, Deal with Angry People, and Living a Life of Mental Wellness and Positivity

Richard Banks

Generalized Anxiety Disorder

Generalized Anxiety Disorder

© Copyright 2021 by Richard Banks. All right reserved

The content contained within this book may not be reproduced, duplicated or transmitted without direct written permission from the author or the publisher.

Under no circumstances will any blame or legal responsibility be held against the publisher, or author, for any damages, reparation, or monetary loss due to the information contained within this book. Either directly or indirectly.

Legal Notice:

This book is copyright protected. This book is only for personal use. You cannot amend, distribute, sell, use, quote or paraphrase any part, or the content within this book, without the consent of the author or publisher.

Disclaimer Notice:

Please note the information contained within this document is for educational and entertainment purposes only. All effort has been executed to present accurate, up to date, and reliable, complete information. No warranties of any kind are declared or implied. Readers acknowledge that the author is not engaging in the rendering of legal, financial, medical or professional advice. The content within this book has been derived from various sources. Please consult a licensed professional before attempting any techniques outlined in this book.

By reading this document, the reader agrees that under no circumstances is the author responsible for any losses, direct or indirect, which are incurred as a result of the use of the information contained within this document, including, but not limited to, — errors, omissions, or inaccuracies.

Thank You!

Thank you for your purchase.

I am dedicated to making the most enriching and informational content. I hope it meets your expectations and you gain a lot from it.

Your comments and feedback are important to me because they help me to provide the best material possible. So, if you have any questions or concerns, please email me at richardbanks.books@gmail.com.

Again, thank you for your purchase.

Introduction 9

Chapter 1- Understanding Your Internal Processes 17

    Patterns of Unhelpful Thinking 20

    Thoughts, Core Beliefs, and Behaviors 26

    Negative Thinking 34

    Summary 37

Chapter 2 - What is Anxiety? 39

    Causes of Anxiety 45

    How Does Anxiety Hold Us Back? 49

    Summary 54

Chapter 3 - Generalized Anxiety Disorder 57

    What is GAD? 57

    Symptoms of GAD 60

    Normal Anxiety vs. GAD 62

    Causes 64

    Diagnosis 65

    Treatment 68

    Summary 69

Chapter 4 - Living with Generalized Anxiety Disorder 71

    Excessive and Uncontrollable Worrying 71

Why do People with GAD Worry So Much? 75

How Can GAD Affect Your Relationships? 78

Overcoming the Stigma 84

Things to Avoid When a Loved One Has Generalized Anxiety Disorder 89

Summary 92

Chapter 5- Strategies to begin tackling physical symptoms 95

Self-care and Relaxation 96

Reducing Stress 97

Brain Food 98

Regular Physical Exercise 99

Spend Time Outdoors 99

Get Enough Sleep 100

Breathing Techniques 102

Summary 103

Chapter 6- Strategies to begin tackling anxiety-provoking thoughts, worries, and cognitive distortions 105

Controlling Your Thoughts 106

Emotional Regulation 107

Mindfulness/ Meditation 108

CBT 109

Summary 112

Chapter 7- Strategies to build confidence and self-awareness 113

   Shift Your Perspective 114

   Mindset 115

   How to Create a Positive Mental Attitude 118

   Augmented Happiness 118

   Become the Master of Your Emotions 119

   Support Network 120

   Summary 121

Conclusion 123

Bonus Chapter 129

   How Your Brain Works 142

   Your Map of Reality 143

   Thoughts, Core Beliefs, and Behavior 144

   Cognitive Distortions 151

   Negative Thoughts 154

   The Role of Trauma 155

   Get Professional Help 161

   Recap 162

Generalized Anxiety Disorder

INTRODUCTION

In the year 2017, it was reported that around 284 million people globally were battling anxiety disorders. Anxiety remains the leading form of mental health disorder. A survey conducted by the World Health Organization showed that 1 in 13 people have dealt with anxiety at some time in their life.

Generalized anxiety disorder (GAD) is a chronic mental illness associated with worrying about minor inconveniences, overthinking about the slightest things, and anticipating worst-case scenarios. People with generalized anxiety disorder are unable to find joy in the little things in life. Concerns about health, finances, relationships, and work are the primary issues that affect people suffering from this disorder.

There's a significant difference between normal anxiousness and generalized anxiety disorder. Normal anxiousness makes us worry about things on a manageable level, but generalized anxiety disorder causes us to be on alert at all times. It keeps us constantly worrying about the minor details of life. Issues of little importance seem to bother the patient with a great magnitude, and they aren't able to help themselves. This type of anxiety brings feelings of hopelessness and helplessness that eat at the individual from the inside. Only the slightest provocation is needed to trigger the anxiousness that comes with generalized anxiety disorder.

Anxiety is a common condition characterized by

stress and worry, and it's often accompanied by obsessive-compulsive disorder (OCD). A person can suffer from OCD and GAD at the same time. People who have OCD tend to remain fixated on a certain issue that bothers them. GAD triggers the anxiety levels associated with that particular issue to a higher degree, making the person more sensitive. OCD patients obsess about things that bother them to the core—like unsymmetric patterns and messes. Anxiety levels go through the roof in a person with both GAD and OCD.

GAD can result from a stressful life. People who deal with stress in their day-to-day lives have a higher chance of being diagnosed with GAD. When they encounter situations that make them feel helpless, this significantly heightens their anxiety levels. Constant worrying is also a contributor to GAD in most patients. This worry often centers on little things in the patient's daily routine that they can't control and that concern and challenge them, including thoughts and beliefs. Over time, constant worrying can trigger GAD.

The constant state of duress in a patient with generalized anxiety disorder is alarming and should be addressed immediately before it worsens. To treat this disorder, patients are prescribed anti-anxiety medications like Xanax and anti-depressants like Zoloft. In addition, patients are advised to go through cognitive behavioral therapy by meeting with a therapist at regular intervals to discuss their issues and deal with their problems in a healthy way. To address generalized anxiety disorder, the patient is advised to change how they live and eat for their betterment. Permanent changes in their lifestyle help them stay on the right track. They're encouraged to take time to meditate, work out, eat a balanced diet, and have a proper sleep routine. Patients are also told to cut back on caffeine and alcohol. Confiding in people close to them is also encouraged to help them feel less burdened by the problems they're dealing with.

If you have GAD, once you get into a lifestyle that's well-suited to improving your mental health, you'll see the difference in the quality of your life, and your worries will diminish. There's no better feeling than being able to take a deep breath and not actively worrying about anything. When you begin cognitive behavioral therapy, you'll find an unbiased listener who will help you work through your issues. Regular workouts and a proper diet will help you feel healthy and happy about yourself and your body. Yoga and meditation will make you feel at peace with yourself. You may be prescribed medication for the short term to act as a bridge as you proceed in the right direction toward better mental health. The credibility of the treatments for this disorder has been established over the years on a global scale. Because GAD is somewhat based on genetics and life experiences, there's no way of knowing if it can be permanently cured. However, it can nevertheless be treated—often successfully. About 43% of GAD patients actively seek treatment, which is a step in the right direction, because you're unlikely to improve if you don't address your situation.

This book will help pave the way to your recovery. The treatment of and the approach to GAD described in this book will make it your go-to guide during this challenging time, and I promise you won't regret giving it a go.

When life throws challenges at you, you shouldn't hide behind a wall trying to protect yourself. You need to go out there and do your best to live your best life. These are challenging times, as the world is battling an ongoing pandemic that's changed our lives completely. The coronavirus has become a huge concern for all people globally and will have a lifelong impact on many of us. Almost all of us have felt some degree of anxiety and stress as a result of this global catastrophe. This paradigm shift has given us plenty of reasons for taking care of our mental health and taking it seriously. Few problems go away just because we stop paying attention to them; we need to face and address them. Reading this book will help you deal with uncontrolled anxiety in unexpected ways.

Generalized Anxiety Disorder

CHAPTER 1- UNDERSTANDING YOUR INTERNAL PROCESSES

How to understand yourself from the inside out

It's said that self-awareness doesn't stop us from making mistakes, but it allows us to learn from them. Every human makes mistakes, but the best attitude is to learn from them. The process may be brutal, but the lesson learned will be a strong one. To know oneself is to know how to live a successful life. People who learn to accept themselves are the ones that find true happiness in life. When you become self-aware, you see things differently. Doors open automatically without you even trying, and life becomes much easier. When you understand yourself, you become accepting of what happens to you as a part of who you are.

To do this, we need to realize that no one is perfect, and everybody makes mistakes. We eventually learn that everyone has their flaws, but those don't make them weak. It just shows they're human. This realization will help you explore many avenues in life. Always enjoy the little victories and celebrate your accomplishments. We feel a sense of achievement when things go right in our life. Leaving your past in the past is the right move. Don't let your past haunt you for the rest of your life, or you'll never be able to enjoy the present moment. Having the patience to deal with yourself will help you go a long way in self-development. Coming to terms with your personality and accepting yourself for who you are is essential. It keeps you grounded and well connected from the inside out.

To understand ourselves from the inside out, we need to understand our past, present, and potential future and accept all of it. When you want to try to have a breakthrough in life, write down your goals and how you plan to achieve them. Living aimlessly will do you no good. Jotting down your thoughts keeps you well connected with your inner self. It also helps minimize the burdens and stresses you experience daily. Get a journal and start writing your thoughts down. This is remarkably effective in working through difficult times. Practicing yoga and meditation will also help you stay calm and composed, and this will help you maintain your mental peace when you face difficult situations in your daily life. Asking questions of yourself will allow you to reach a deeper understanding of who you are. When you come to terms with your personality traits and flaws, you'll be one step closer to understanding how they shape your life—including your life going forward. Once you understand your inner and outer life, you'll be able to use these superpowers to assess other people and make better life decisions. When you improve yourself and learn from your mistakes, people around you won't take advantage of you.

Also, understanding yourself has a direct effect on your mental health. When you know yourself, you can take charge of your life situation. When you're in control, you thrive.

Patterns of Unhelpful Thinking

When people cling to the negative aspects of life, they fall into a pattern of unhelpful thinking. When things don't go as planned, people may feel hopeless and helpless, which can trigger worry, stress, and anxiety to an excessive degree in people suffering from GAD. For example, say you're stuck in traffic, and your mind starts to wander into the deepest, darkest places in your life. You start coming up with the worst possible scenarios of how things will go down. This is an automatic response to any type of stress or disaster happening in your life. Before you know it, you're spiraling down.

We can't entirely control what we think about and how we deal with it. More than half of the time, the mind wanders to places where all we can see are the bad things in life. When you let these negative thoughts get the best of you, that's when you can start losing yourself to GAD. The constant pressure of stress might pull you down and cause a great deal of distress, but the key is not giving up and letting it take over your mind.

One way to deal with these unhelpful thought patterns is to learn how to work with them. If something that hasn't even happened yet is troubling you, you need to learn to let it go and not let it occupy a large portion of your mind. There are plenty of significant and important things in life to worry about, so the slightest inconveniences shouldn't upset your mental peace. When you stop inflating these minor issues, you'll learn to prioritize and deal with problems in a much better way.

You also need to be able to distinguish between what's real and what's not. Going through a setback in life might pull you into your usual unhelpful thinking patterns, but you need to lift yourself up, dust yourself off, and get back in the game. Nothing good is likely to be delivered to you on a silver platter; we have to work for all good things in life.

The following is a list of unhelpful thinking pattern symptoms:

Catastrophizing

Catastrophizing is when the problem you're dealing with is of small magnitude, but you blow it out of proportion and make it into something so massive that it overtakes your mind. When a single piece of negative information is given to you, and you make a big deal out of it, that only makes things worse for your mental health. When you think of things negatively, you won't find solutions for them, and you'll become stuck in a loop. See things for what they are, and try not to make a fuss about them.

Jumping to conclusions

When life is going smoothly, no one knows what's going to come next. The healthiest way to live it is to wait for things to unroll on their own, sit back, and watch the show. When you try to take control of the outcome, that's when things go wrong. When a person with GAD believes they know something is going to happen, they'll automatically assume the worst possible outcome.

When you look around at a gathering of people, study their expressions, and make quick judgments about what those people might be thinking about you, this is also a sign of unhelpful thinking patterns. When you're quick to make assumptions about what will happen in the near future, you'll ruin your ability to appreciate what's happening currently.

Overgeneralization

Something happened in the past, and you cling to it for so long that you start applying the same formulas to events in the present or events that might occur in the future. This is an unhealthy thinking pattern that needs to be stopped. Dealing with different situations in a similar manner isn't the right way to go about it. Every circumstance has its own complexities and should be dealt with on its own terms.

Mental filter

When a person is suffering from a mental health disorder, they focus on the negative parts of the situation at hand. A negative mental filter focuses on the negative aspects of the situation and completely ignores the positive parts. This makes your mind focus on the negative patterns in your life. Accepting the situation as a whole will help you help yourself.

Maximize and minimize

When we maximize another person's traits and minimize our own, this can negatively affect our mental health. When we suffer from low self-esteem, we tend to think better of others than of ourselves. Our sense of self-importance is diminished if we keep doing this. Seeing the good in people is one thing, but completely belittling yourself is an act of unhelpful thinking. We may also come up with reasons to make our achievements look small. This is also unhealthy for our self-esteem, so we need to take credit where we deserve it.

Irrational emotions

When your anxiety is driven purely by emotions, you know you're spiraling downward. Something hasn't even happened, yet you anticipate that it *will* happen and it won't go well. This is an unhelpful thinking pattern. It gets you stuck in a frame of mind that won't let you move forward in life. When you don't handle a situation based on logic and let your emotions take control, your suffering increases.

Thoughts, Core Beliefs, and Behaviors

Your thoughts, core beliefs, and behaviors make you who you are as a person. Your beliefs, perceptions, and experiences construct your thoughts. Your outlook on the world helps you become self-aware. When your knowledge is limited, your thoughts about a particular topic are confined within those limitations. To break those barriers, you need to broaden your mind. Your thoughts can eat you alive or make you successful in life. Sometimes, you can control what you think, but, at other times, you have no control. Usually, it's the latter. It's on you to decide where you want to invest your time and your thoughts. Your thoughts and behavior arise from your core beliefs.

How are beliefs formed?

Our core beliefs are usually developed in childhood—to a great extent by our parents. They expect us to learn and practice what they teach us. Those things help establish our morals and principles in life, and these help us live a grounded life and become a better person. As children, we naturally look to our parents and older siblings for guidance. Our surroundings also help us build the palace of our mind, which we furnish with our thoughts.

How we look at the world is dependent on our core beliefs. They're often associated with our life experiences. What we went through in our past and what we're going through right now affect those core beliefs. If we've witnessed something in our past and have made up our mind about it, it becomes hard for others to change our perception and core beliefs. Sometimes, what others tell us becomes the truth we start believing in. For instance, whatever our elder sibling tells us about the world when we're a child may form our beliefs about it.

Our relationships also have a strong impact on forming our core beliefs. Sometimes, our belief system is linked with our perceptions of the world and things happening around us. Factors that affect our core belief system can be both internal and external.

Our natural temperament also plays a huge role in our beliefs. Certain things aren't suited to our character, so we don't believe in them. Changing our core beliefs is like changing how we think about ourselves. It's difficult and time-consuming, but if we make up our mind to change these beliefs, we'll alter them once and for all. Of course, all of this depends on our mental strength and how much we can take on. When we start questioning our beliefs, that's when we'll be able to put a stop to our unhelpful thinking patterns. If we don't put a stop to them, they become an endless, painful loop.

Differences between thoughts and beliefs

On a lazy Sunday afternoon, your mind wanders to different places when you stare at the blank wall in front of you. Your mind is full of thoughts, and there may be a thousand things going on at the same time in it. A person with GAD tends to focus on certain thoughts and obsess about them. Every thought doesn't have the same weight in your life and your mind. The thoughts that have the most weight are your beliefs. If a thought has the power to change your mind stream and affect your life decisions, that surely means it's something you believe in. A belief is a thought that you accept with all your heart and mind.

A chain reaction we can follow to differentiate between a thought and a belief begins with a thought that creates an emotion that leads to you taking action based on it. That, in turn, leads to a result. To prove that the result is right and what you're feeling is correct, you need to review the result repeatedly before forming a belief about it. After your belief system is established, you can take a back seat and let your belief system generate your thoughts automatically. Thoughts induced by your belief system ultimately influence your behavior.

The role of perceptions in how we think

A perception gives your thoughts a direction, which is how the two are interlinked. Your thoughts about a particular topic interpret the information you gather with your senses. This gives you something to ponder, which might result in a change in how you think and act. Perceptions are the reality of life. Each person has their way of thinking. Each person reacts to the same situation differently, but how you respond to that situation reflects your perception of that thing. When we try to dig deeper into how and why people think the way they do, we gain some understanding of people's perceptions toward different things. Each person reacts differently than every other person, and there's always a reason why a person behaves the way they do.

How you behave in the presence of others is also based on your perceptions. For instance, if you start thinking that your best friend is becoming distant because you haven't been spending as much time with her/him lately, you'll naturally behave distantly when you meet her/him. That's because you've set up a particular perception about that person. As a result, you'll feel a change in your behavior and temperament when dealing with that person. This misperception can cause a lot of problems between the two of you.

A perception not only controls how and what you think about, but it also affects how you see the world around you. It's like a bubble that you've built around yourself, and you're moving within it.

Merely thinking a thought may not immediately change your core beliefs, but those thoughts can form new beliefs over time through repetition. In the long run, thoughts may also be able to change your reality as well. They aren't able to change your situation, but they may be able to change who you are as a person. They might equip you to deal with a situation in a much better way. You're in charge of how you feel. If you allow your mind to have happy and contented thoughts, you will be contented with life. Otherwise, you'll always see yourself as a victim of your situation and your thoughts. Your thoughts are powerful enough to change your life and your situation. Negative overthinking will make you immensely miserable. The endgame is to study your thought patterns and intercept your thoughts when they become negative.

Cognitive distortions

Cognitive distortions form a pattern of negative thinking that's usually based on an incorrect and negative bias. We might "adjust" the facts and figures of a situation, knowingly or unknowingly. We might blow something out of proportion because our mind has set up boundaries and made decisions, and there's no changing them. We might assume the outcomes of things that haven't even happened, and we might start acting on those assumptions. We tend to forget the fact that for something to go wrong, something has to happen first. Where there's no smoke, there's usually no fire, which might be hard for some overthinkers to understand. People might make a situation worse than it is by overhyping and exaggerating the event in their minds. Sometimes, when we overcomplicate things, we find ourselves stuck in that loop of negative thoughts with no way out. In a way, cognitive distortion causes our minds to convince us of something that isn't even true. This may result from past events, and the urgency to jump to conclusions might not go away quickly. To overcome this, you must be dedicated; the process takes time and effort.

Negative Thinking

Negative thoughts are a result of thinking about something that deeply disturbs or scares us. They're the opposite of the natural stream of thoughts that flow through our minds throughout the whole day and sometimes change our mood. Negative thoughts often afflict a person going through a bad phase in their life. For instance, a sick person might only have negative thoughts going through their mind all day long as they lie in bed. To disrupt that stream, they need to be distracted by having something else to focus on. A person who's having a busy day might also fall into a negative thought pattern that might take a toll.

When you identify your negative core beliefs, you become self-aware and self-critical. This gives you an opening to become a better version of yourself. But, unfortunately, these negative thought patterns might hinder your path by discouraging you from reaching your full capacity and living up to your expectations and hard work.

There are several reasons underlying the tendency to think negatively—not having a high regard for yourself, believing you're not good enough, believing you won't be able to do something, having the idea that trying to do something would make you look stupid, wondering if your life has no purpose, believing a particular thing that you want to do is too difficult for you to handle, and believing you have no options. These are the kinds of negative thoughts that hold you back and become an obstacle on the road to success.

To restructure your negative thoughts, you need to start working on yourself. You need to find ways to calm yourself so your anxiety level isn't hitting the roof. You need to find the root cause of what triggers your anxiety and creates negative thoughts. You might be able to tackle your anxiety better if you jot down your negative thoughts and find ways to eradicate them from your life. You need to make an effort to understand why you think what you think. This will give you a better understanding of everything in your life. You also need to accept criticism aimed at your betterment by viewing it as constructive and helpful in allowing you to grow out of your negativity.

To stop these thought patterns, you might look for distractions like shopping, playing games, self-care treatments, and keeping your loved ones close to you. You need to make sure that you appreciate the good things in life because they don't come around often. Negative thinking is just a waste of time and energy. It's not worth spending half of your day worrying about things that might not even happen, or, even if they do occur, what's the point of worrying about them beforehand?

Summary

All in all, to understand the internal processes, you need to focus on yourself and what you believe in. Once you start organizing your thoughts, you will be able to control your mind and your actions. When you are in control, you don't get anxious very often. Your feelings shape your thoughts, and your thoughts construct your perceptions. Your behavior and your core beliefs are a part of that system. They help in creating your outlook towards the world. To keep your mental health on the right path, you need to rid yourself of the negative thinking patterns and cognitive distortions that will hinder your path and creativity.

CHAPTER 2 - WHAT IS ANXIETY?

What exactly is anxiety?

Anxiety is a feeling of unease, such as worry or fear, and the symptoms range from mild to severe. Some people can become anxious after a specific, identifiable event, such as a trauma. Anxiety is the body's way of responding to stress. It's what we feel when we're put into what we assume is a threatening situation. Anxiety is also an umbrella term that covers several diagnosable conditions, which we'll explore further. Anxious thoughts and feelings are perfectly natural for everybody from time to time, but it becomes a problem when we experience anxiety that's persistent, seemingly uncontrollable, and overwhelming.

Anxiety causes us to feel nervous and uncomfortable. It might be triggered by fear of a particular thing or anything that's not in our control. Anxiety levels vary from person to person. For instance, on your first day of college, you might feel awkward sitting in a room full of new faces and interacting with those people. This can lead to anxiety.

When a person feels anxious, their body can become tense, and their responses can become urgent. You might become oversensitive about the slightest inconveniences and look at things in a different light. Anxiety clouds our thinking and, most of the time, an anxious person doesn't make the wisest decisions. Anxiety is an overwhelming feeling that gets the best of you and your judgment. It mentally upsets you and makes you impulsive, or, in some cases, it makes you incapable of making decisions. It slows down your reflexes and makes you worry over the slightest details. It stops you from living a normal, happy life. It intrudes on your mental peace and doesn't let you make good life decisions.

Some common misconceptions about anxiety can give people the wrong impression about the seriousness of this mental disorder and even create a societal stigma around anxiety. People might stop taking you seriously, and patients who need treatment might not seek professional help because of the stigma of admitting that their anxiety affects their lives. The stigma discourages people suffering from anxiety from coming forward with their issues and voicing them as a way to find relief. The misconception that anxiety can be dealt with logically is false. We can't expect a person with anxiety issues to explain why they react in a particular way. If we think they're unaware that some of their worries don't make sense, we're wrong. Anxious people are aware of how silly some of their fears may seem, but that doesn't stop their worrying.

Anxiety isn't just in our head; it can affect our body as well. Our body might get triggered by a string of negative thoughts that are disturbing our mental health. In some cases, anxiety can lead to heart problems. It can also cause physical symptoms like sweating, nervousness, panic attacks, and much more. People with GAD experience anxiety round the clock over long periods, which is very different than people who occasionally get nervous.

Another misconception is that every person has the same reaction to their GAD; everyone has their way of responding to and dealing with things that cause anxiety. For instance, if a person has nervous sweats when he gets anxious, that doesn't mean that another person with GAD will nervously sweat when in a similar situation. Finally, anxiety shouldn't be confused with depression. It's common to confuse anxiety with depressive behavior. Anxious people have a string of thoughts about how things could go wrong and out of hand, while people suffering from depression primarily have negative thoughts about their lack of control in life and feel they're stuck in that life with no way out.

Where does anxiety come from?

As Khalil Gibran once said, "Our anxiety does not come from thinking about the future, but from wanting to control it."

When you suffer from anxiety, it can seem like nothing is under your control. The more fearful you feel of not being in control, the more you try to structure your world to feel safe. Perhaps you had previous experiences with feeling powerless, and you never wish to feel that way again. To address this, you may overcompensate by exerting significant control over your current environment, including the people around you. You try to control all the details of the events occurring in your life that disturb your mind, and you lose focus.

Anxiety affects everyone at some point in their life. However, it can affect some people more than others, to the point where it becomes disabling. Most people don't recognize their anxiety for what it is and instead think there's something "wrong" with them. Some people are preoccupied with the symptoms of anxiety (e.g., stomachaches, increased heart rate, shortness of breath, etc.) without realizing the cause. Others think they're weird, weak, or even going crazy. Unfortunately, these thoughts only make people feel even more anxious and self-conscious.

As awful as it can be, anxiety is a normal part of life that can arise at any time. Even if you don't have an anxiety disorder, you've probably experienced anxiety at some point. To effectively manage those emotions, you need to understand where the root cause lies by identifying the causes of anxiety.

Causes of Anxiety

There's no one cause of anxiety because every case is different. However, many people experience overlap in their anxiety symptoms and causes. Below are some of the common sources of anxiety:

Genetics

Some people suffering from anxiety have it in their DNA. It usually runs in their family, so they're more likely to be affected by it. Their genetic predisposition causes them to get upset over petty things, and their fight-or-flight mode gets triggered. This is inherited from generation to generation, and there's not much you can do to change it. If you have blood relatives that have been diagnosed with an anxiety disorder, there's a higher chance of you getting diagnosed with it.

Past traumas

Abuse has become a sad reality of the world we live in. People are abused and harassed in their homes, their workspaces, and in public settings. If a child witnesses a disturbing scene, they tend to hold on to it for the rest of their life. If they're abused or harassed, this forms a lifelong memory as well. The memories of that event will haunt them for the rest of their life in the form of anxiety and other mental disorders. Anything that deeply affects us lingers. Children who've been subjected to abuse and trauma are also victims of anxiety. The same goes for people who've been traumatized as adults. A person's circumstances have a direct effect on their mental health.

Fighting an illness

When you're undergoing treatment for or fighting a serious illness, it's a process that's rife with worry, and that affects your thoughts, daily routine, and almost everything in your life. You're scared for yourself and how things will turn out, and so are the people around you. This makes you worry about the situation even more. Not being able to tell what the future holds for you or if you'll survive this illness prevents you from sleeping peacefully at night. This worry becomes the root cause of your anxiety.

Personality

Some people naturally have a personality that makes them easy prey for anxiety. For example, people who have a submissive nature are more likely to fall into a pattern of anxiousness than people with a dominant character. People who are overachievers and perfectionists tend to become easy targets for anxiety as well. Thus, your personality plays a huge role in the likelihood of falling into anxiety.

Upcoming event

Hype about an event or situation in your life might also cause anxiety. The buildup before the actual event doesn't make the clock tick faster. It may be an event you're really looking forward to, but the waiting is excruciating. For example, whenever you're about to go on the podium to give a big speech, you feel anxious before that walk-in moment. This is entirely natural because of the adrenaline rush in your body before a big event. When you overhype things, it makes you even more anxious and also affects your overall performance. It doesn't matter if that event is big or small; the anxiety can still disable you.

Substance Abuse - Drugs and Alcohol

The misuse of drugs and alcohol is also a leading cause of anxiety. If you're already suffering from anxiety, these two can make things even worse for you. Alcohol and drugs can trigger and exaggerate your emotions and send you into a loop of negative thinking patterns and places you don't want your mind to go to.

How Does Anxiety Hold Us Back?

If we don't address our severe anxiety, it will hold us back in life. Anxiety tends to inhibit our productivity and positive thoughts, and it interrupts our day-to-day activities. Our suffering is amplified when we feel anxious and we're unable to think straight. Anxiety creates a feeling of helplessness and hopelessness, which can be terrifying. The anxiety that you're suffering from can take a significant toll on you. It might affect your relationships with the people close to you. It might affect the quality and quantity of your work, making you lag behind in your workplace. It might affect your health. It might occupy your mind throughout the day, making you incapable of experiencing and doing good things in life.

Anxiety holds us back in several ways, including:

Losing self-confidence

Your self-confidence allows you to reach your full potential. If you don't have self-confidence, you won't be able to accomplish all of your goals and dreams in life. When you don't have self-confidence, you stop believing in yourself, and, eventually, others around you stop believing in you, which can hurt you deeply. Anxiety preys on your self-confidence and diminishes it, so you lose touch with your inner self. Stress and worry lower a person's self-esteem, making them feel weak. In a room full of successful people, they'll feel like a misfit because they believe they're not good enough to be in that room standing with those people. This, in turn, causes them to lose faith in themselves. We lose our ability and will to work hard and do what we want to in life. When we lose our self-confidence, we tend to hide in other people's shadows. We stop fighting for our place in the world, and in return, we often don't get credit for all the work we did. When others give their opinions on our lack of self-confidence, that tears us down even more.

Overwhelming fear

When anxiety overcomes us, we feel a kind of overwhelming fear at all times. This feeling doesn't go away, and it keeps affecting our life. There can come a time when the crippling anxiety and uncontrollable fear won't let us leave our house or even our bed. Our will to do anything is lost. Individuals who are dealing with anxiety find it difficult to look for opportunities and interact with people. It can affect a person's finances, social life, personal life, and professional life. Once all of this is gone, the person may lose their will to live as well.

Missed opportunities

To make it big in the world, you need to take chances, and chances involve risks. The person who's willing to risk everything is the one who takes chances, and that one right choice might help them become successful in life. It's all about the right decision at the right time. But, for people dealing with anxiety, it's tough to experiment with new things and opportunities. They prefer to do something they're familiar with because they want to eliminate the risk factor. For such people, significant accomplishments rarely happen. They're slaves to normalcy and old patterns; thinking out of the box isn't for them. Lesser opportunities mean lesser success, and this is where the problem lies. You might not get the promotion in the first run, but you might get an upgrade if you take advantage of the right opportunity at the right time. It's all about taking chances and being dedicated to accomplishing your goals.

Lack of interest

When we're anxious, we don't feel like being a part of things that are outside our comfort zone. If a person suffering from anxiety doesn't feel like socializing, they'll skip their boss's party and maybe miss out on the once-in-a-lifetime opportunity to get a promotion. Our lack of interest in things might make us the least favorite person in the office. We don't interact with anyone in the workplace, and that makes us the odd one out. We aren't a part of any of the office squads, and we aren't invited to our coworkers' house parties. This lack of social interaction makes us feel miserable at some point, but we're too stubborn to admit it. The lack of interest in participating in office gatherings throughout the day, only thinking about the end of the shift all day long, and not being part of anything major in the office can prevent our career from taking off.

Not adhering to deadlines

Jobs are based on getting work completed before the deadline. An anxious person will have high stress levels whenever a deadline is approaching. This often paralyzes them as the deadline looms closer. They may even be unable to complete the work, but this is beyond their control. They're the victim of their anxiety. They're unable to get the job done on time, and, as a result, they may miss their deadlines—which, of course, reflects poorly on them. They may be let go on and miss out on learning new skills and having new experiences. They taint their image in their boss's eyes, and this usually doesn't turn out well for them.

Summary

Anxiety is an overbearing feeling that weighs on your mind and body and makes you unable to carry on with your day-to-day activities. It occupies your mind and stops you from being productive. Discouraging people who have anxiety issues might make them stay stuck in this zone for life, and generalizing all the people with this problem doesn't do them any good. Not knowing what the future holds for you is an uneasy feeling for people with anxiety. Anxiety holds you back from living a normal life and being social. Anxiety disorders are different types that might trigger panic in a person such as, selective mutism, separation anxiety, generalized anxiety disorder, panic disorder, and many more.

Generalized Anxiety Disorder

Chapter 3 - Generalized Anxiety Disorder

What is GAD?

Generalized anxiety disorder creates excessive worry and uncontrollable anxiety about any number of things. The people who suffer from GAD can ruin things for themselves by anticipating chaos and downfall. Even if something good comes their way, their anxiety causes them to ruin it for themselves. Many things can trigger anxiety in people with GAD—their relationships, family, work, finances, health, and many others. They don't need valid reasons to start worrying and overthinking. Even the slightest inconveniences make them feel like their world is collapsing. Sometimes, there might not even be a trigger for their constant worrying—it just happens without a cause. People with GAD don't just have anxiety once in a while; it regularly occurs over a long period. When this happens, it's necessary to take it seriously before it too late.

Women tend to be affected by GAD more than men. There's no usual onset age for GAD patients, and it may differ for each person according to the events going on in their life. There are no specific causes in people who are diagnosed with GAD. Still, over the years, a pattern has been observed in people with a family background of GAD. People living in a stressful environment and who aren't doing well in their lives are more likely to be diagnosed with GAD. People who are dealing with GAD symptoms find it tough to go through the day without breaking down.

They find it impossible to be productive and creative and accomplish quality work. They often procrastinate and end up wasting their day. They lag in work, and the work setting can become unbearable for them. Sometimes it's obvious to them that what they're worrying about poses no real danger, but they still can't help worrying about the outcome.

People with GAD tend to try to control situations by meticulously planning every detail, but, in life, things often don't go as planned, and that upsets them to the core. GAD doesn't only affect them mentally but can create physical symptoms like a stomachache or headache, which only make them feel worse.

The functionality of people with GAD varies from person to person. Sometimes a diagnosed person might be able to participate in social gatherings and thrive at their workplace. Others might not have the energy to carry out the simplest tasks. It all depends on how their symptoms affect their energy throughout the day. GAD can also make some people feel restless or even panicky.

However, there are effective ways to deal with GAD.

Symptoms of GAD

A person diagnosed with GAD may show any of a variety of symptoms. These symptoms range from mild to severe, depending on the person. The symptoms can be physical or psychological. A person might manifest just one symptom or several.

The physical symptoms of GAD include tiredness, heart palpitations, shortness of breath, acne or other skin problems, allergies, stomachache, headache, dizziness, drowsiness, lethargy, sweating, nervousness, vomiting, nausea, shaking, muscle aches, insomnia, and many more, all of which make the patient's life difficult.

Some psychological symptoms include a sense of dread, lack of focus, irritability, restlessness, and constantly becoming annoyed over little things. These symptoms can make the individual intolerant and unable to cope with new or difficult situations in their life.

If you're a person with GAD, it can directly affect your behavior as you go through your daily life. To put a stop to these overwhelming feelings, you might begin to think that cutting off social contact with people you hang out with is a good idea. You start canceling on people you're close to and start bailing on plans with your friends, family, and colleagues. This will put you on the outs with everyone who makes an effort to stay in touch with you, and they may quit trying after your sudden behavior change. You might lose the people who genuinely care about you by shutting them out of your life like that. It can make you constantly stressed, which might also affect your self-esteem, making you feel even anxious.

Normal Anxiety vs. GAD

Distinguishing between everyday anxiety and GAD can be tricky. So how do you know, especially if you tend to be a little more anxious than other people, whether or not your anxiety is significant enough to qualify as a disorder?

We all worry and experience some degree of anxiety due to relationships, deadlines, careers, and finances. However, people with GAD experience persistent, excessive, and unrealistic worry that goes on every day—and possibly all day. They feel their anxiety is beyond their control and they always expect the worst, even when there's no reason for concern.

Normal anxiety can become severe if it's not managed properly. It can take a huge toll on your daily life, making you unable to carry out your work efficiently. It will lower your work production and make you lose out on greater opportunities.

However, GAD is much more severe than normal anxiety. It's possible to have some control over normal anxiety, and there are a number of methods for doing this. People with normal anxiety may find techniques to calm their nerves, but these aren't effective for individuals with GAD. People with GAD have a hard time remaining calm throughout the day; they aren't able to stop stressing over the minor details of their life.

People who have normal anxiety become anxious in situations with a high degree of worry and urgency, but the situation doesn't get exaggerated in their mind. However, people with GAD overhype the situation and make it something more significant than it is.

Normally anxious people are affected by anxiety for shorter periods, and their anxiety level is usually milder. In GAD patients, the anxiety level is intensified and lasts for a more extended period. When people experience normal anxiety, they tend to become anxious over specific things that make them scared or nervous, like attempting an exam or giving an interview. On the other hand, GAD makes a person anxious all the time over everything. This is what distinguishes GAD from normal anxiety. Both are of equal importance, and they should be treated appropriately to prevent them from getting worse.

Causes

The causes that lead to a diagnosis of GAD include a family history of this mental health disorder. People who suffer from GAD usually have a predisposition to it in their genes, making them vulnerable to the disorder. People who've had a traumatic past also fall prey to this disorder. When people are put in stressful situations, they tend to become victims of constant worrying, and, over time, this makes them fall into a pattern characteristic of GAD. For instance, if someone close to them is going through a stressful treatment for cancer, they're likely to get caught up in worry because of the uncertainty of the success of the treatment. People who are subjected to abuse as a child are more likely to be diagnosed with GAD.

Childhood traumas stay with us throughout our lives and can make us feel vulnerable and sensitive over time. The pain we've been through reappears in bits and pieces—sometimes as flashbacks—and it doesn't allow us to move on with our life. Excessive usage of caffeine or tobacco also makes us an easy target for GAD, and continuous usage can make the condition worse.

Diagnosis

A mental health professional or a doctor can diagnose generalized anxiety disorder in patients in several ways. The person must be evaluated at a clinic or hospital. If you're feeling relentless, overwhelming anxiety, you should head straight to the doctor and get examined. The doctor will do a thorough physical check-up to determine the cause of the anxiety. It's possible that it's a side effect of a medication or the symptoms of an underlying disease. The doctor will do a detailed evaluation to rule out other possible disorders to determine if the diagnosis is GAD.

There will also be laboratory tests such as a complete blood panel to determine if there are underlying physical issues. Your doctor will then ask if you have a family history of this illness or if you've had other episodes in your personal history. Next, to ensure an accurate diagnosis, the doctor might ask you to fill out a psychological questionnaire and evaluate your responses to determine the nature of your anxiety. Finally, the doctor will use medical directories to cross-reference the responses to assure you do indeed have generalized anxiety disorder.

A person with generalized anxiety disorder will display one or more of the symptoms of the disease for at least six months. The long duration of symptoms is what differentiates this disease from normal anxiety. GAD is characterized by severe anxiety over a long period of time. A person with GAD is unable to control or deal with stress and or any kind of challenging issues in their life. They may obsess for minutes, hours, or even days about the slightest details of their life that may hold no or little importance in a normal person's life. They over-examine things to an extreme degree and typically find little joy in anything.

Several symptoms occur in a person suffering from GAD, but most patients diagnosed with the disease have three or more of the following symptoms:

1. Episodes of the mind going blank and brain fog

2. Ongoing lethargy
3. Being edgy and getting annoyed easily
4. Being restless
5. Continuously missing deadlines
6. Muscle pain and body aches
7. Unable to sleep

The discomfort and dread caused by these symptoms might make it difficult for the patient to function properly in normal settings. In addition, these symptoms keep them distracted and detached from their everyday life, making them miserable while doing routine tasks. If you have GAD, it's essential to be diagnosed and treated, as this will significantly improve your chances of having a normal life.

Treatment

Generalized anxiety disorder is an extensive, long-term ailment that, without treatment, can plague patients for years or even most of their life. However, there are several treatment options for this debilitating disorder. The specific treatment prescribed depends on the person's response since each person's symptoms and severity are unique.

There are two main approaches to the treatment of generalized anxiety disorder. One is the use of medication, and the other is therapy. Both of these are effective, but deciding on the type of medication or therapy is dependent on the person, their symptoms, the severity of their disease, and their response to the treatment.

Summary

Generalised anxiety disorder is a mental disorder that causes you to worry about everything at an alarming level. It has physical and psychological symptoms that include dizziness, lethargy, loss of appetite, lack of focus, inability to carry out daily activities, and many more. GAD is different from normal anxiety because of its severity. The diagnosis can be carried out by mental health professionals that will do a thorough check up on the suspected patient. The treatment for GAD can be done by the use of home remedies, by self-help, by psychotherapy and by medication. The seriousness of this disease should not be questioned, and it should be looked into before it's too late.

CHAPTER 4 - LIVING WITH GENERALIZED ANXIETY DISORDER

Excessive and Uncontrollable Worrying

An English proverb states, "Worrying is like sitting in a rocking chair. It gives you something to do, but it doesn't get you anywhere." Generalized anxiety disorder is like sitting in that rocking chair and wasting the whole day doing. Nobody can deny that good and bad things happen to us all the time, but when we let the bad stuff overtake our thinking, we fall into ongoing anxiety. Once anxiety gets the best of you, you'll find it very hard to overcome it. Winning the battle against anxiety is a slow and lengthy process, but you have to trust the process if you want it to be successful. Worrying excessively and uncontrollably doesn't get you anywhere.

Living in the moment should be our goal in all stages of our life. If you constantly plan, and nothing goes according to those plans, your mental health may fall into shambles. Life isn't always fair. It has its ups and downs, and you have to move forward without complaining because there's nothing you can do to undo the damage that's already been done. It's better not to waste your time regretting things that can't be undone. In the long run, when you worry excessively, you may try to control all aspects of your life. This is usually unsuccessful, and that further negatively impacts you. There are times when you aren't even sure if the events you're anticipating will occur or not, but you exhaust yourself mentally worrying about them beforehand. All this does is destroy your peace of mind.

Negative thoughts are endless, and they can take up most of your day. A day that could be spent on something productive is wasted on thinking about things you can't control. This not only exhausts you mentally but also exhausts you physically. It may go on for minutes or hours; it's like a loop of thoughts constantly overlapping and making a mess in your mind. You come up with events that might not even happen, but imagining them makes scenarios in your mind, and you think about them anyway. These are the first thoughts you become aware of when you wake up, and they're the last things on your mind before you go to sleep. You find yourself thinking about what might happen when you're having your food or reading your newspaper or even when watching television or conversing with someone. You easily zone out of conversations. You may start missing deadlines, and you can no longer produce quality work, making you feel bitter about yourself. Suddenly, it's not about proving to others that you're good enough; it's about proving it to yourself.

The more you think about whatever it is, the more you become invested in it. The more time you spend thinking about something fools you into thinking it's the right way to go about it. You might start believing that thinking about it over and over will help you look at things in a different light. You become fixated on the idea that procrastinating and overthinking might help you find new ways to deal with whatever it is. So you rely on excessive worrying and overthinking to guide you in the right direction. As a result, the worries and tensions might start dominating you, giving you less and less control of your life over time. It starts with one thing, and that leads to something else, which leads to another thing. It's an endless loop of worries that never go away if you let them take over your mind.

You start overthinking about all the aspects of your life, making it way worse for you. Telling yourself you can't help it or you've just accepted this as a part of your life isn't a valid excuse. People who help themselves are the ones that are deserving of help. If you don't make an effort to pull yourself out of this negative thinking, it's highly unlikely that it will go away on its own.

Why do People with GAD Worry So Much?

When we get done with a stressful episode and reflect on our actions, we usually regret the part where we worried about things too much. Eventually, all the worries go away—all the concerns that did nothing but take up a lot of your time and consume a lot of your energy. The key is not to let it pull you down.

At a time of peak stress, people don't realize to what extent worrying too much ruins their life. It costs you your precious time, your energy, your social standing, your relationships, your finances, your family life, your health, and your professional life as well. Most of the time, what we worry about never happens. It's just in our head, which doesn't let us get over things easily. It can't be denied that the future is uncertain, and there's nothing humanly possible that can help us control what's coming toward us. Some people are under the impression that bad things don't usually happen to people who worry too much. That's a myth and has no reality or facts to support it. When you worry too much, you lose your peace of mind. People think it's helpful to anticipate all the worst-case scenarios before the actual event so they won't be blindsided when something terrible happens. It gives you the feeling that you're equipped to handle anything bad that comes your way. You don't realize it takes up a lot of your mental function and time to keep you prepped for the bad times. You can't really plan how to deal with problems before they happen, and you need to make peace with that. Getting blindsided isn't the worst thing that could happen to a person.

Living in the moment helps you stay calm about what the future holds for you. People also start believing that if they worry too much, it means that they care more. Caring about something and getting upset as a result of worrying too much about that thing are two different considerations. A definite line has been drawn distinguishing the two.

Sometimes people think that worrying too much motivates them to get their work done. The argument is that people who are laid back find it difficult to get their work done on time compared to people who worry a lot and get things done on time because they're afraid of the consequences they could face if they didn't get it done on time. They like to believe that worrying makes them creative and productive, but there's no truth to this. Worrying only makes you preoccupied, so you can't focus entirely on the problem at hand.

How Can GAD Affect Your Relationships?

People suffering from generalized anxiety disorder often struggle in many aspects of their lives, including in the relationships department—relationships with your family, partner, friends, and even your colleagues. When your worries have an overbearing effect on you, it takes a toll on your relationships with people close to you. If people use negative thinking to make life decisions related to their relationships, this usually results in a strain on those relationships. When you struggle with feelings of anxiety about yourself and the people around you, it puts a lot of pressure on your relationships. This is because of the way you start looking at things in your life. The change in your approach makes you a different person in the relationship. Negative thoughts usually evolve into negative feelings and negative experiences. You might start second-guessing the nature of your relationship; how things will turn out between the two of you, how you'll manage things, what your boundaries are, or whether the relationship will last. You might ask yourself if this is the right person for you, should you look for other options, is the person loyal to you, is this a balanced relationship, are you capable of keeping the other person happy, and does the other person make you feel happy? These are the sorts of questions that people with GAD often have about their relationships—sometimes on a daily basis.

When you're dealing with problems related to GAD, and you're also investing your time and energy in a full-time relationship, you may start becoming insecure about where you stand with that other person. You might start having doubts about your importance in the other person's life. No matter how much validation the other person gives you, it might not satisfy you to the point that you become content with it. You start doubting your significant other's feelings for you—or if they ever loved you to begin with. You might start thinking that maybe that person doesn't want you to be around them, or they might want to take a break or break up with you. All of this will only lead to sabotaging your relationship with that person. No matter how hard they try to make you feel good about yourself, you'll be stubborn enough not to listen to them.

There are times when you risk destroying your relationship due to your anxiety issues, and you might not even be aware you're doing it. When you start having relationship problems due to GAD, this goes on to create issues for you such as not allowing you to pay more attention to your relationships or be expressive. You may be impatient about things, and have low self-esteem, self-confidence, and trust issues. You might be irritable in a relationship rather than being in the moment and enjoying it. You may act awkward around people, not responding with the right reactions at the right time, feeling overly dependent on the other person, expecting too many things are that are unreasonable, or feeling insecure.

Maintaining a relationship is always difficult. It's a two-way street where both people must contribute to make it work. If one of the partners stops contributing, that's when problems arise. A successful relationship requires both partners to be expressive, communicative, trusting, truthful, patient, caring, understanding, and loving. The other person feels a sense of security and affection when you try to be all these things. When a mental disorder like GAD affects your mental health, you start struggling in many of these areas of your relationship. There's a good chance that your partner or the person you're close to might not know how to deal with your anxiety. They might say something that upsets you, but they shouldn't be held accountable if anything goes wrong. It should be understood that this is your battle, and no one else can help you with it if you're not willing to help yourself. When you become overly dependent on the other person, the burden of the relationship automatically shifts onto that person.

A person is used to carrying their baggage, but when a person with GAD dumps their baggage onto the other person, it becomes unfair and puts a strain on the relationship. You rely on your partner for constant support and validation, but when the water goes over the bridge, that's the right time to bail out. Nobody wants to over-invest in something they don't believe in anymore.

Sometimes people with GAD tend to become detached from the person they're close to. These two extremes—putting the burden of maintainting the relationship entirely on your partner or, conversely, detaching yourself from them—are game-over for a relationship. The ignorance of the importance of the person you're in relationship with can make you distant from them. For the most part, it's on you and your partner to deal with GAD and try to cope with it to keep your relationship alive and well. You need to realize that your partner isn't your unpaid therapist who's obligated to listen to you ranting all day long.

There are professionals who do that sort of work, so you should never burden your significant other with something they don't know how to help you with. It will only make them feel worse to think they're not able to help the person they love. You also need to understand that they aren't your rehabilitation center, so you need to start working on yourself without expecting someone else to come along and fix you. This approach will only make you stay stuck in your mind's anxiety zone.

It's a good idea to be open about your issues with people you trust and ask them for advice about how you should handle things. Advice from someone we're close means a lot to us and gives us an extra push improve ourselves. You shouldn't overwhelm your partner with a constant stream of emotions. They should be given the right to decide to what extent they should be involved in your journey. If your partner is working on themselves, you should be the first person to help and encourage them on this path. And if your partner is having difficulty with what you're going through, encourage them to get professional help for themselves. Whether we like it or not, a relationship has a lot of effect on a person dealing with GAD.

Overcoming the Stigma

Generalized anxiety disorder is a disease commonly found in people dealing with severe anxiety issues. Do you blame the person diagnosed with cancer for putting themselves through this ordeal and making them think it's all in their head? There's a stigma associated with generalized anxiety disorder, and it's this lack of awareness by society that's been the biggest obstacle for people dealing with GAD. This stigma often stops them from seeking professional help and may result in the deterioration of their mental health.

People diagnosed with this disorder have a hard time fitting into society because of this social stigma. Patients with GAD tend to believe they won't be socially acceptable if they expose their issues to others. They have a fear of not being accepted by other people. They are often cruelly labeled as "psychopaths" or "insane" by society, making them feel uncomfortable when they're in a social gathering. People need to understand that mental health disorders aren't a personal choice. Harsh assumptions will only make people with GAD feel insecure and diminish their self-esteem.

Most people view a person with GAD quite differently from a normal person. Those who are dealing with the issues related to the disorder feel embarrassed and helpless when people around them don't take them seriously. The stigma attached to this issue impacts the health of the person with GAD. Their mental health starts deteriorating because of the excessive pressure to be "normal," which is called "societal pressure." Around 40% of people globally have been impacted because of this stigma, and it's stopped some of them from getting help. Embarrassment can keep people silent about their struggles for a long time, and this demoralizes them. Not being able to vent or share your struggles with someone is perhaps the worst aspect of all. You feel you can't seek wise advice because you're too afraid of being judged.

People with GAD may become easy targets for bullying and harassment. People try to take advantage of their insecurities and their weaknesses, making them feel bad about themselves. They struggle with having fewer opportunities in the job sector. Their friends and family misjudge them, and they become sidelined. People seem to have little sympathy or even the ability to understand that no one wants to feel miserable and lose sleep overthinking and excessively worrying about something not in their control. No one wants to remain lonely and become a slave to their negative thoughts. No one willingly wants to feel they can't control their emotions. It should be stated loud and clear that no one wants to live like this and that educating people about GAD is the most helpful way to assist someone struggling with this condition.

To overcome this stigma, people who don't suffer from this disorder need to school themselves and educate others. Do research to understand the facts fully. You need to understand all the characterstics of GAD so you can help your friend and not make their life more miserable than it already is. You should be aware of how you behave and what comes out of your mouth when interacting with a person with GAD. You should reflect on any of your problematic opinions before voicing them. When you know the root of the problem, it's easier for you to understand how to deal with it and how to help your friend. You need to choose your words wisely so you don't cause offense. When you feel you've educated yourself enough, make sure that others around you are also aware of how to deal compassionately with people suffering from GAD.

We need to treat everyone with respect and show decency to encourage and motivate others to come forward with their struggles so they can get the help they deserve. We should make everyone feel included, especially people dealing with GAD. Being understanding makes them feel safe and improves their self-confidence. The discrimination that people with GAD deal with daily hurts them to the core. People with GAD shouldn't be ostracized by their disorder. They should be known for who they are. To help with this, they can join support groups to make them feel better by interacting with other people dealing with similar issues. They might also think about speaking up about their issues on a larger platform that will help others as well. When we empower people with GAD, they feel listened to and that they matter.

Calling out the people who do you dirty is another form of self-empowerment, so don't let anyone tell you that you're not good enough. If you're self-sufficient, that's enough to make them stop bothering you. This is another approach that can be implemented to overcome the stigma linked to GAD.

Things to Avoid When a Loved One Has Generalized Anxiety Disorder

When there's someone in your life who's been struggling with generalized anxiety disorder, you need to make them feel empowered so they know you're there for them through thick and thin. This makes them feel important and cared for. Even when you're trying to be considerate, there are times when you might have a slip of the tongue or when you're indifferent to the critical situation that person is in. To avoid that and not make the person with GAD feel bad, you need to be mindful of certain things when dealing with that person. Don't tell them to stop overthinking or excessively worrying. They may be offended by this because you should know they can't help their behavior.

There are many things you can say to be supportive, such as, "I'm here for you," or "What can I do to make you feel better?" Don't try to solve their problems for them. That might not be helpful and just add to the problem without you knowing it. Just be present as they work through possible solutions. Sometimes, the other person only wants you to be there and sit quietly. Just being there and not saying anything can make a lot of difference. When you try to solve their problems and take on their burden, it can make them feel they're useless and incompetent. They may begin to feel they can't do anything right, which will make things worse for them.

The last thing a person with GAD needs to hear is, "You should be grateful that something worse didn't happen to you." Most important of all, don't lose your patience when talking to a person with GAD. Talk to them softly, and try to sympathize with their problems, not add to them.

The following are statements that shouldn't be said to a person with GAD:

- "It's not that big of a deal."
- "Why are you overthinking it?"
- "Why are you getting anxious because of it?"
- "I know what you're going through."
- "Just breathe."

- "It's all in your head; you're worrying about nothing."
- "Get over it."
- "Just stop thinking about it. "

These are the wrong things to say to a person with generalized anxiety.

Summary

When you have to live with generalized anxiety disorder, excessive and uncontrollable worrying becomes a part of your life. It ruins your life and occupies most of your valuable time. Worrying is normal, but it is seen as a major red flag that needs to be looked into when it becomes a part of your daily routine. People with GAD worry so much because they find it very hard to stop once they start thinking. They obsess over the slightest issues and go over the details repeatedly that makes them anxious at all times. They like to control their future and know what will happen beforehand, so they fall behind.

GAD has a negative effect on your relationships because excess baggage weighs on the equation you have with your significant other. The stigma related to anxiety disorders hinders the path of people struggling with it. It makes them silent, inexpressive, uncomfortable and lonely. To overcome the stigma, you need to make this as normal as possible by educating people around you, encouraging the people with GAD to come forward, and many more approaches in the right direction. Things that you should avoid when someone very close to you is diagnosed with GAD are being overly efficient and trying to solve their problems, not being supportive, not having the patience to deal with their issues and much more. To live with GAD is a very difficult journey that can be made easy if you have the right people to support and encourage you.

Generalized Anxiety Disorder

CHAPTER 5- STRATEGIES TO BEGIN TACKLING PHYSICAL SYMPTOMS

When a person is going through a rough patch in life while struggling with GAD, he/she is a target of not only psychological but physical symptoms, such as headaches, heartaches, stomach ache, nausea, sweating, palpitation, and shaking. To tackle these physical symptoms, you need to take some steps in the right direction. Some of the steps are mentioned below:

Self-care and Relaxation

When you are diagnosed with generalized anxiety disorder, it becomes a significant part of your life. Most of your day will be full of worries and constant stress. To take a break from the fiasco, you need to make sure that you spend your time in self-care and relaxation. To break the circle of negative thoughts, you need to spend time with yourself. It will work like a distraction from your ground realities so you can calm your nerves. Everyone deserves a me-time where they can do things that make them happy and at ease. For example, you can go to a salon to get a manicure or a pedicure done or get a facial, so it will make you feel better about yourself. For relaxation, if you are reading books, you can start reading novels of your preferred genres and even self-help books that will help you. Self-care and relaxation do not take away your anxiousness, but they act as an escape for them. And sometimes, it is the only thing that matters.

Reducing Stress

When you have a lot going on in your life, you need to take some time out to reduce your stress level. The constant grind will leave you exhausted physically and mentally. You are the only one who can break that stress cycle to give yourself a much-needed break. There are several ways to relax. For instance, you can light up a candle and read your favorite book while lying down on the couch. You can watch your favorite movie. You can binge-watch a show that you've been planning to watch for so long but never got the time to watch it. Surprisingly chewing gum is something that calms your nerves and keeps you distracted. If all of this does not help you tackle your physical symptoms, you can reduce your caffeine intake. You can also choose to start journaling by writing down what you feel at that moment. You should also take out time to spend with friends and family, have a great laugh, and get an escape from your physical symptoms of GAD.

Brain Food

There are supplements available in the market that can help you deal with the physical symptoms of GAD. The Omega 3 supplements work as brain food and are known to reduce the symptoms by 20%. It improves your heart health and keeps you healthy. Other supplements like St. John's wort elevates your mood and makes you less lethargic throughout the day. And 5-HTP is another amino acid supplement that produces serotonin in the body. Vitamins (B and D) are also helpful in tackling the physical symptoms of GAD. They make sure that your body is functioning properly and overcomes your body weaknesses due to GAD symptoms. Vitamin D especially takes care of your bones, muscles, and your teeth. Supplements and other brain food will ensure that they minimize the intensity of the physical symptoms by a considerable amount.

Regular Physical Exercise

As Reese Witherspoon once said, "Exercise gives you endorphins, and endorphins make you happy." It shows that physical exercise plays an integral part in keeping your mental health intact and reducing GAD's physical symptoms. There are a few reasons why and how working out helps you tackle the physical symptoms of GAD. Such as it helps you in lowering the release of stress hormones. By following a workout routine, you get habitual to a healthy lifestyle that will keep your mind off negative thoughts and the physical pain that comes with it. Regular workouts help you in developing a stronger body and nervous system. It also enables you to build a better image of yourself, which in return helps build up your mental health and get you rid of issues that pull you down.

Spend Time Outdoors

With your eyes shut, soaking in the heat on a bright sunny day is all it takes for you to relax. Staying indoors, tucked in your bed all day long, or sitting on the couch watching television or playing Play Station won't get your nerves to calm down. For people dealing with GAD, this is an epic escape from realities. Sunbathing gets your mind off things and allows you to take it all in. when you shut your eyes, you realize that all the worries in your life are vanishing, and the pain in your body due to anxiousness is fading away. That is the moment you live for, and that is what it takes for all the sadness to vanish at the moment. You should realize that it is okay to take some time out for yourself and just be with yourself away from the noise of the world. Spending time outdoors will allow you to acknowledge the beauty of nature, and it will give you moments of relief when you finally get to have a break from all the reality checks that have been haunting you for quite a while.

Get Enough Sleep

Just as your body needs food as a fuel to function,

your body also needs enough sleep for you to operate properly. As science suggests, a person needs an average of 8 to 9 hours of sleep daily. This is an adequate amount of sleep that will help you re-energize your body and keep you fresh. When your body does not get the time to relax while sleeping, it tenses and becomes rigid. That tension in the body causes the physical symptoms of GAD to worsen. To overcome the symptoms, you need to make sure that your body relaxes and takes its fair time. When you oversleep or under sleep, your mind and body stop coordinating with each other, making you mess up everything you put your mind on. Going to bed on time will allow you to fix your routine and keep you running through the day. Good sleep will improve your attention span and focus on things that matter in life. So to tackle the physical symptoms of GAD, getting enough sleep is integral.

Breathing Techniques

When you feel overwhelmed by the anxiousness, you need to try breathing techniques to help you breathe properly and help make you feel better physically and mentally. First, you need to lie down on whatever is right in front of you and comfortable enough to lie down peacefully. Next, shut your eyes for a while and let it all sink in. When you breathe through your nose with your mouth closed, you need to keep breathing for 6 seconds. Ensure you don't take in too much air in your mouth at a time, or else it will become overbearing for you. Exhale for another six seconds as your body relaxes and your lungs settle down. You need to repeat these breathing techniques for at least 10 minutes so you can finally calm down. Make sure that your jaw and your cheekbones are relaxed. Finally, you should let go of your body so you can fully relax. After a while, you will see immediate results that will help you feel better.

Summary

Certain strategies that will help ease the physical symptoms of GAD are self-care and relaxation that will help you get your mind off things so you can focus on yourself. Reducing the stress you are feeling is of foremost importance, do things that make you happy. It will create an escape for you from reality that will make you feel better. Brain food is essential in the proper functioning of the body. When you work out regularly, it helps you build up an excellent routine to overcome your physical symptoms. Spending some time outdoors in the sun will help you get some me-time that you very well deserve. Getting enough sleep is necessary for your body to operate. Some breathing techniques help you in calming your nerves down. All of these should be practiced to overcome or at least minimize the physical effects of GAD.

A Short Message from the Author

Hey, are you enjoying the book? I'd love to hear your thoughts!

Many readers do not know how hard reviews are to come by and how much they help an author. I would be incredibly thankful if you could take just 60 seconds to write a brief, even if it's just a few sentences!

Thank you for taking the time to share your thoughts!

Chapter 6- Strategies to Begin Tackling Anxiety-Provoking Thoughts, Worries, and Cognitive Distortions

It is completely normal to deal with anxiety in times of stress. Sometimes it is the presentation in front of the whole that is causing it, and sometimes it is the idea of getting married to someone. But when those episodes go from rare to very often, things go South, and it becomes a serious problem to your health. As a result, specific strategies are followed to minimize the anxiety-provoking thoughts, cognitive distortions, and worries that allow you to grip your mind.

Controlling Your Thoughts

When you can control your thoughts, you get a hold of your life, which is how you can turn your life around. Controlling your thoughts is in itself an art that is not very easy to master. The first step to control your thoughts is to be prepared and staying one step ahead. When your mind is ready to be hit with setbacks, the damage control unit in your brain does not allow anxiety to rush into your system. Understanding that fear will only hinder your way and slow you down is another step in the right direction. Do not let your fears control you and define you. When you stay grounded and in touch with your realities, your thoughts do not stray from the path of positivity. Staying and living in the moment will help you narrow down your thoughts, which will cut down the negativity in your life. Speaking your negative thoughts aloud will guide you in not getting in over your head whenever you face an obstacle. This is an effective strategy that will help you eliminate anxious thoughts, cognitive distortions, and unnecessary worries.

Emotional Regulation

To stay positive in life, emotional regulation is necessary. Human beings are hungry for information and insight into what's going on in the news and around them. The more they get to know, the more they get desperate to get hands-on new gossip. It is a basic human instinct, and it cannot be tamed if you don't shift your focus on things that will help you build yourself in the long run. If you start working on yourself and try to get to know yourself, you will regulate your emotions more efficiently. When you find yourself in a situation, your behavior will reflect how you think about your situation. So when you are stuck in a dire situation, you need to keep calm and not do anything impulsive. When your mechanism comes back to normal, you should then take action. When your brain detects negativity around you, it automatically responds to it and builds a coping mechanism. For regulation of emotions, you need to channel your thoughts to take control of your responses. When you feel that something is going wrong around you, you should try to focus on things around you and how they make you feel. Try focusing on the five senses and how they are affecting your surroundings at that moment. By accepting the situation and being understanding about it will show you the right way for emotional regulation.

Mindfulness/ Meditation

Once you start meditating and get used to that kind of peace, your mind will automatically find ways to dig deeper into the peace every time you meditate. It takes you in the zone of your mind where you feel like all your stress and worries have vanished. There's nothing but you and your escape from reality that calms your nerves. You tend to be happier and relaxed when your mind is at peace that means no negative anxiety-provoking thoughts running around. Mindfulness and meditation help you deal with the negative thoughts that have been bothering you. It guides you to cope with all of it and live your best life. It not only improves your sleep cycle but also maintains your diet. As Jon Kabat-Zinn said, "You can't stop the waves, but you can learn to surf." It shows that you might not control what happens to you, but you can always find ways to tackle what disturbs you mentally and physically. And that is where mindfulness and meditation come in. Mindfulness helps you savor the moment you live and enables you to cherish it while it lasts and sometimes after it. And meditation gives you an escape route and calmness that is so much needed in a stressful life.

CBT

Cognitive-behavioral therapy is a kind of

psychotherapy that deals with mental health problems like anxiety, depression, stress, and drug problems. It helps you figure out your life's purpose and helps you restructure your negative thoughts, and give them a push in the right direction. In generalized anxiety disorder, cognitive behavioral therapy has been known to do wonders for patients. It allows the patients to break free of their unhelpful thinking patterns and challenges the cognitive distortions that twist and turn your thoughts. It also eliminates your negative core beliefs.

Certain negative core beliefs lower your self-esteem and pull you down in life. Cognitive-behavioral therapy helps you recognize your self-worth and helps you live with your flaws by accepting them. CBT also guides patients in connecting their thoughts to their emotions and how they behave. It channels your negative thoughts into positive thoughts and makes sure that you can better assess each situation.

Understanding destructive behaviors is a way to know the thinking patterns of a person you are dealing with during CBT. The past is not of great value while undergoing CBT; the center stage is given to your life's current and future events. It is also to ensure that you do not put yourself in harm's way when dealing with something that can have a negative impact on your mind. Sometimes the destructive behavior is subjected to others around you or even to yourself. The purpose of this psychotherapy is to make sure that it doesn't happen.

The ABC model is a technique that is used by mental health professionals when they are performing CBT. The concept of an ABC model is that the behavior and emotions of a person are not necessarily based on the events that occur but on how you interpret or process those events and emotions. The activating event will lead you to start believing in something that will control the consequences of how you think and act. This is how CBT deals with your thoughts and helps you in finding the right direction in life.

Summary

The strategies mentioned in this chapter are essential to tackle anxiety-provoking thoughts, worries, and cognitive distortions. They will enable you to control your thoughts by getting your life together and knowing what to react to and how to react to certain events. Emotional regulation will keep you composed while dealing with a stressful situation. Mindfulness and meditation will allow you to live in the moment and not think ten steps ahead. In this way, your mind will stay peaceful in stressful situations. Finally, cognitive behavioral therapy is an effective method to tackle negative thoughts as it works on restructuring how you think and deals with situations that might provoke you.

CHAPTER 7- STRATEGIES TO BUILD CONFIDENCE AND SELF-AWARENESS

Self-confidence is what makes you strong in situations that pull you down. When you start believing in yourself, the world starts believing in you. Everything falls into place automatically when you give yourself a chance. Self-awareness gives you the confidence to carry your flaws, like making you who you are and are comfortable in your skin. It shows that the anxiousness you are feeling will go away when you do not let it affect you from the inside. Second, guessing your self-worth is what makes you weak in moments like these. So some strategies to build your confidence and self-awareness are as follows:

Shift Your Perspective

Fixing your behavior and shifting your perspective will help you build confidence and gain self-awareness in life. It is your decision about how you want to perceive your thoughts. You are the one to decide how your thoughts will impact your outlook towards life. You have the power to choose whether your thoughts make you feel good or bad when an event or situation occurs. You make your own choices, and there is always something better than the negative options. It helps you decide what you want for yourself, and this is how it helps in believing in yourself. When you take responsibility for your actions, emotions, and perspective, it gives you a sense of confidence and makes you in control. Being in the driving seat of your life is what keeps you going in the right direction. When you lay in bed, you should go through everything significant that happened throughout the day; it will give you a review of your day, which keeps you from repeating the same mistakes. A new and reformed outlook towards life changes how you see the world and helps you eliminate anxious thoughts and worries.

Mindset

Reviewing your way of thinking

Reviewing your way of thinking is like rewiring your brain before it self-destructs and results in making bad decisions in life. When you keep your thought process in check, you make sure that you make wise decisions for your good. Thinking your way to getting better confidence skills will help you get what you want and feel good about yourself. Life is a game of how strong your mindset is. When you think before you speak or take action, you are on the road to recovery.

Taking action

Do not let yourself sulk in a puddle of emotions. If you want to take control of the reigns of your self-confidence, you need to put a stop to your negative thoughts before it's too late for you to get out of it. Pull yourself and dust yourself off and get back in the saddle. Convince yourself to do it and make sure that you don't overthink any of this. When you take consistent steps in the right way, you will be able to make sure that you see its end. Eliminating the distractions from your path is also another way to get the work done on time.

Positive mindset

Positive things happen to those who have a positive mindset. When you think negatively, negativity tends to follow you wherever you go. Manifestation is a way of believing that good things will happen for you until they start happening in actuality. Think positive so that it helps you build your confidence to the point that you see the good in yourself and others around you. It makes you a better person in the eyes of yourself. Having a positive mindset will help you deal with things better because it will give you optimism even if things don't go as planned.

Self-awareness

Knowing your realities and where you stand in life helps you in becoming aware of yourself. It helps you in investing more time and energy in yourself which ultimately boosts your confidence. Self-awareness helps you in improving your skill set and correcting where you lag. It also works with you to handle your emotions, not mess up your work and personal life. Keeping a balance between the two is what helps you keep your confidence on high levels. When you are self-aware, it gives you the power to practice what you are good at and gives you a reality check on where you need to improve.

How to Create a Positive Mental Attitude

To create a positive mental attitude, you need to focus on the things you are grateful for. Counting your blessings will help you become self-aware and humble. When you funnily see things, it makes it easier for you to deal with the difficult times. Surrounding yourself with positive people who correct your mistakes and motivate you to become a better version of yourself is the kind of people who will help you create a positive mental attitude. Identifying your areas that need work is another way of raising your self-confidence and awareness.

Augmented Happiness

The science of happiness tells us that it is not only the good things in life that make you happy, but it is how you see the world and what you think is good for you is that makes you happy. Similarly in augmented happiness, where you convince yourself what is good for you and what is not, decides how happy or miserable you are in your life. When you convince yourself that whatever you have right now is enough for you, your mind automatically accepts it and goes easier on you. It is the ultimate goal for every human being to be at peace with him/herself which whatever he/she has. And when someone is genuinely happy, it reflects in their personality and how they carry themselves.

Become the Master of Your Emotions

A confident person will be able to identify his/her emotions right away. The key to becoming the master of your emotions is not to suppress them or be in denial about them but to accept them and use them in a way that paves your way to getting what you want in life. The emotions could become fuel on the road to achieve your ambitions. Processing your emotions fully before you act on them helps you in practicing self-control. Raising your emotional intelligence will help you become aware of your roots and the roots of others around you. Ensure that you don't make bad decisions in the heat of the moment, and identify what triggers your negative thoughts and emotions. That will help you get a grip on your emotions.

Support Network

A support network is a group of people that push you to be better and achieve your goals in life. They encourage you to adapt and perform well in life. The ones that care about how you are doing in life are your support network. They help you with your social skills, which is a big factor in your confidence building. They help you in coping with negative thoughts and behaviours. They help you in elevating your self-esteem by making you feel good about yourself. The feeling of completeness when you are with them helps you to succeed in life. When you are with them, it feels like the world is at your disposal, and everything is made easier for you.

Summary

Several strategies are to be followed if you want to build your confidence and self-awareness. Shifting your perspective to have a positive outlook towards life is one of them. Working on your mindset to get a better grasp on things is another. Reviewing your way of thinking will help you learn from the mistakes you've made in the past and not repeat them. Taking action will help you get things done on time. A positive mindset ensures that good things happen to you. Self-awareness boosts your confidence and lets you work on the aspects where you lag. Creating a positive mental attitude will help you perceive things differently, which allows you to think out of the box. And augmented happiness will guide you in becoming content with where you stand in life. Becoming the master of your own emotions will allow you to become aware of how you feel about things. And a support network is the group of people that push you to do better in life and feel good about yourself.

Generalized Anxiety Disorder

Conclusion

The message of this book is that generalized anxiety disorder is a serious mental illness that must be addressed with great care and dedication before it becomes a grave problem that takes over your body and mind. You should seek treatment so it doesn't get worse and you can start to enjoy your life again. You need to step up and bring your A-game to tackle it.

All around the world, people deal with anxiety on a daily basis. However, constant and debilitating anxiety shouldn't be left unchecked. It might eventually take away your will to live. Facing your problems is the first step in overcoming them.

This book offers several methods for relaxing and avoiding stress that will allow you to have healthier responses to the challenges in your life. It also explains how your emotional well-being is greatly affected by your thoughts. Third, it will guide you in putting an end to your unhelpful and negative thinking patterns and thought processes. Fourth, it will allow you to come up with steps to address your anxiety. Finally, it gives a detailed account of how cognitive behavioral therapy works in your favor by allowing you to look at things differently.

For people who want better mental, emotional, and physical health, this book will help you in all of these departments. Generalized anxiety disorder affects your overall well-being and greatly impacts your mental clarity and self-confidence. This book will guide anyone who's willing to work on their emotional needs, self-awareness, and happiness.

Understanding how your mind works is what gives you an inside look at your thinking patterns. The life of a person struggling with generalized anxiety disorder is different and more complex than an average person's life. They have to deal with physical and psychological symptoms that make life more challenging than it already is. The strategies put forth in this book to deal with the physical symptoms outline an escape route from the anxiety you face regularly. Techniques are discussed that will allow you to control your anxiety-provoking thoughts, worries, and cognitive distortions. The steps to build your confidence and become aware of your will are designed to allow you to see a stronger person when you look in the mirror. All of this will help you manage your generalized anxiety disorder so it takes a back seat in your life.

The premise of this book is to provide a detailed account of generalized anxiety disorder to give you a better understanding and awareness of a disease that affects many people globally. GAD has made a considerable impact on the death rate around the world. This book promised to help you in dealing with dire situations and get yourself out of them. Putting an end to anxiety was the sole purpose of this book, and it contains everything you need to practice calmness of mind and lessen your anxiety. The solutions are explained thoroughly—from mindfulness and meditation to shifting your outlook toward greater positivity. Everything has been covered to give you a better understanding of what you're dealing with.

The one thing I want the reader to take away from this book is that you can become self-confident. This is key when you're struggling with generalized anxiety disorder. Self-confidence not only makes you self-aware but also grateful for all the blessings in your life. It allows you to deal with situations in a much better way when you believe in yourself and what you stand for. Don't let life and your circumstances push you down. If you don't help yourself, others around you won't be able to help you.

All in all, this is a complete guide to assist you in working through your anxiety and emerging into mental freedom.

One more thing

If you enjoyed this book and found it helpful, I'd be very grateful if you'd post a short review on Amazon. Your support does make a difference, and I read all the reviews personally so I can get your feedback and make this book even better. I love hearing from my readers, and I'd really appreciate it if you leave your honest feedback.

Thank you for reading!

BONUS CHAPTER

I would like to share a sneak peek into another one of my books that I think you will enjoy. The book is titled **_"How to Deal with Stress, Depression, and Anxiety: A Vital Guide on How to Deal with Nerves and Coping with Stress, Pain, OCD, and Trauma."_**

Are you tired of wasting your time and energy worrying all the time? Do you see the irrationality of constant worrying, but you can't seem to stop doing it? Are you ready to learn how to deal with anxiety and depression without taking drugs?

This book will walk you through precisely why, how, and what you need to do to stop worrying and start living your life.

Nearly 800 million people worldwide experience mental illness. Some of the most prominent adverse mental conditions include stress, anxiety, and depression. These can lead to recurring periods of sadness, worry, anxiety, loss of vigor, loss of interest, poor concentration, and feelings of worthlessness. These issues can affect your psychological and physical health, and when you let them go untreated, they can have longstanding effects on your life and relationships. The more you ignore your mental strife, the harder it becomes to be resilient in the face of hardship, and if you let emotions get out of hand, they can lead to increased mental illness.

Though stress is an inseparable part of our lives, we can easily manage it using simple strategies and techniques. All we need is the willingness to learn these techniques and the ability to take action. Effective stress management is critical to your physical, psychological, and emotional health. It's vital to your overall well-being. This book will show you how to start managing your issues and get relief immediately.

How to Deal with Stress, Depression, and Anxiety provides a complete framework and a well-rounded set of tools to understand the causes of stress, depression, anxiety and how to overcome it.

Enjoy this free chapter!

Generalized Anxiety Disorder

Virtually all people experience stress, anxiety, or depression at various points in their lives. One 2017 study suggested that about 792 million people worldwide have formal mental health disorders, with depression and anxiety being the most common conditions. Millions, maybe even billions, of additional people experience subclinical conditions and high levels of stress, so the number of people who deal daily with such issues is quite astounding. When you live with any of these conditions, everyday activities become a challenge, and you may resort to self-sabotaging behaviors, or you feel stuck in place.

As these conditions continue, it only makes you feel worse, both mentally and physically. In the United States, it's been reported that stress affects the mental health of 73 percent of the population, leading to worsening conditions like depression and anxiety. While these conditions are all too common, they don't have to be. Living with mental illness or stress can feel impossible, and that's a hard burden to carry, which is why mental distress often leads to further mental and emotional anguish.

The Challenge

With so much external pressure in today's society to be their best selves, millions of people worldwide struggle to maintain their mental health and professional or personal well-being. Many emotionally and physically harmful behaviors—such as overworking and extreme self-sacrifice—are glorified by society. As people are pushed to do their best work and make room for a personal and social life, they can become consumed by anxiety and worries that impede their progress.

The statistics on stress, anxiety, and depression depict a grim picture. As the most prevalent mental health issue in the United States, according to the Anxiety and Depression Association of America, anxiety impacts over 40 million American adults, representing over 18 percent of the population. Globally, nearly 300 million people have anxiety. People who have anxiety tend to have greater stress levels, and 50 percent of those diagnosed with anxiety will also be diagnosed with depression. Depression rates are also startlingly high, with just under seven percent of the population experiencing major depression at any given time and another two percent experiencing persistent depressive disorder, also known as dysthymia or chronic depression.

Even if you don't have a clinically diagnosed issue, such as depression or anxiety, you likely have some degree of stress that makes it harder to function as you'd like to. The Global Organization for Stress says that 75 percent of people are moderately stressed, and nearly all people experience stress at some point in their lives because of a myriad of contributing factors. With so much mental dysfunction, it's no wonder that some people think they'll never get better, but this grim picture doesn't have to be your reality.

While mental health conditions have the power to destroy and debilitate people—paralyzing them and making it hard to have hope for the future—there are proven techniques anyone can use to improve their mental health and allow greater opportunity for personal development. You do not need to let your stress, anxiety, or depression hold you back anymore.

The solution to managing your mental health isn't easy or quick, but it is effective. With effort and careful attention to a multi-faceted plan, you can make dramatic improvements to your damaged mental health and start investing more energy into things that make you the most gratified. There are several steps you must follow for the best results. When you apply these steps, you can have increased mental clarity, emotional freedom, and confidence. Curing your mental health issues will require you to face everything that scares you and to admit uncomfortable truths. Still, you'll be far better off when you seek help than the nearly 25 million Americans who have untreated mental health conditions. You may not need the same level of care as people with more severe conditions, but you do need help because living with any degree of stress, anxiety, or depression is living with more pain than you need to have.

Treating a mental illness can seem intimidating to many people, but there are several effective methods, and there are ways to treat, if not cure, any mental health condition you may have. With so many adults and children not currently being treated for their mental health issues, it's no wonder that mental health statistics remain so prevalent. Still, with increased awareness and the greater availability of mental health resources, the prognosis for those who have mental illness continues to improve. Alongside this, as these issues become more widely acknowledged and discussed, the stigmas attached to them are beginning to dissipate, which removes some of the shame linked to mental illness, which only exacerbates it. Accordingly, by committing bravely to treatment and opening yourself to increased understanding of mental illness, you create resilience against mental illness and become more proactive in the treatment of these debilitating conditions.

For those of you with any of these issues, you cannot delay treatment. Mental dysfunction of any kind makes it harder to feel joy and, in the worst cases, it can deprive you of your ability to function. More than that, your mental health can also impact your physical health. For example, research has shown that stress increases the chance of someone dying from cancer by 32 percent. The Canadian Mental Health Association says that people with poor mental health are more prone to having chronic physical disorders.

A study from Johns Hopkins University found that patients with a family history of heart disease were healthier when they engaged in positive thinking. Among the participants of the study, those who had a positive outlook were 13 percent less likely to experience a cardiac event. Additionally, they found that, generally, people who have better outlooks live longer.

The Solution

Recovery is a process that isn't always linear, but this book will lay out the basic steps to help get you on the right track. The first step in the process is all about education. Before you can do anything else, you must understand the beast you're trying to slaughter and the sword you'll use to slay it. You'll learn how the brain works and how problems with its wiring can lead to mental dysfunction. You'll also learn how you can rewire your cognitive processes to promote increased mental health.

In the second step of the process, you'll continue your educational journey and gain a more in-depth understanding of what anxiety, stress, and depression are and how they impact the way you function. You'll start to understand how to address each of these issues using essential coping tools.

Once you've learned about each condition, you'll be introduced to one of the most powerful psychological tools for improved mental health: Cognitive Behavioral Therapy (CBT). You'll discover what CBT is and how to use it to address your mental ailments.

Once you understand the founding principles of these conditions and the fundamentals of CBT, you'll learn how to manage your circumstances daily by overcoming roadblocks and reviving your sense of self by shifting your perspective as you begin to think in new ways. You'll start to care for both your body and your mind in life-changing ways. All of these steps will lead to mental clarity and mental liberation.

With all this in mind, it's clear that a person's mental health impacts every part of their life, and without addressing your mental dysfunction, you'll never have the peace of mind you crave. Each day you do nothing about your mental health is another day you deprive yourself of health and happiness. Your mental health should be your priority, because you cannot fully function as a member of society if you're prohibited from doing all the things you love the most.

If you feel like you are losing sight of yourself and your desires because of your stress, anxiety, or depression, it's time to make a change. It's okay to be nervous about the adjustments you will need to make to feel healthier, but remember that being uncomfortable and uncertain is vital because they represent change. If you don't change, you'll never feel better than you do now. Maybe you have learned to live with your pain and worry, but it's time to learn to live without those negative coping mechanisms because they stop you from living your life to the fullest.

While the techniques in this book can help you improve your levels of stress, anxiety, and depression, I recommend seeking professional support to help push you towards your goals.

There are tons of books on this subject on the market, so thank you for choosing this one! "How to Deal with Stress, Depression, and Anxiety" will provide a complete framework and a well-rounded set of tools for you to understand the causes of stress, depression, anxiety and how to overcome it. Please enjoy!

How Your Brain Works

Too many people hurt their recovery journey by working against their minds. They think they can force their brains into submission, and when that doesn't work, they feel like failures. When a change you're trying to make doesn't stick, it is usually because it isn't one your brain is used to. As much as you may want that change, your brain will resist it because unfamiliar things feel unsafe to the human brain. The human brain loves patterns, and it uses those patterns to create your internal mental programming and perceptions of reality. When you understand how your brain works, you can use it to your advantage to create new patterns and reframe your mental state.

Your brain is a powerful force, and it can work in remarkable ways. In facing your worries, doubts, and other negative feelings, you need to understand how your brain functions so you can stop fighting your brain and start working with it.

Your Map of Reality

In 1931, scientist and philosopher Alfred Korzybski established an important metaphorical notion with his statement, "The map is not the territory." He believed that individuals don't have absolute knowledge of reality; instead, they have a set of beliefs built up over time that influence how they perceive events and situations. People's beliefs and views (their map) are not reality itself (the territory). In other words, perception is not reality.

Your brain fills gaps in understanding automatically. This means that when you don't know something, you subconsciously make an estimation based on the information you do know. When you experience worry or sadness, this can be caused by a map of reality that reinforces those ideas. That worry or sadness lingers in your mind and can shape future decisions unless you reshape your perception. Your map of reality will always be an interpretation, but it can be an interpretation that helps you rather than hurts you. You can change your map of reality and make it more productive by addressing your thoughts and beliefs and how they impact your behavior.

Thoughts, Core Beliefs, and Behavior

Beliefs are sets of ideas that individuals use to dictate how they'll behave. A belief is something you think is a fact. You feel so strongly about something that you're almost positive it's true, regardless of how well you can prove it. You may have some doubts from time to time, but, overall, you consistently stick to those beliefs. Beliefs are attitudes that you fall back on, because they provide a sense of security, and they make you feel that certain things are constant, which is why something that makes you doubt your beliefs can be so painful. Your beliefs drive your unconscious, habitual behaviors. They become so ingrained in you that they feel natural and inherently true.

When you have trouble managing situations or coping with feelings, you automatically turn to your beliefs for help without exerting too much brainpower. Your beliefs help you determine morality, and they help you decide whether people or things are bad or good. Your whole perspective uses a compilation of your beliefs to fill in the parts of your reality you can't fully understand.

Beliefs are formed based on past experiences and the stimuli around us. Most people's core beliefs—the most driving beliefs they have—are established when they're young children. As they grow older, children commonly challenge the beliefs they've been taught as they begin to think more critically and independently. Nevertheless, many children reaffirm the beliefs they were taught rather than disproving them. As adults, they can challenge these beliefs and, by managing their beliefs, they can create a healthier view of the world that's a more realistic map of reality.

Beliefs can be incredibly powerful. For example, imagine parents telling their children that paperclips are dangerous. Telling a child that paperclips are dangerous seems silly. Nevertheless, when those words go unchallenged, the child will internalize the message, and they might try to avoid paperclips, which could impede their ability to do certain tasks. But as they grow older, the child would likely challenge that belief and overcome the fear of paperclips.

Other beliefs may be harder to debunk. For instance, if a mom tells her child that dogs are dangerous, the child may become afraid of dogs. This fear could continue into adulthood, because the child has learned to be terrified of dogs. Even rational arguments that dogs aren't something to be scared of may still make it hard for that child to believe. After all, dogs, unlike paperclips, do have the potential to bark and bite. The child would be so convinced by the belief that it would be hard for them to break from that mindset.

You may have beliefs that stand in your way and feel so foundational to who you are that challenging them makes you uncomfortable. Nevertheless, you need to contemplate your limiting beliefs.

While thoughts and beliefs may seem similar, there are some profound differences between them that you must acknowledge if you want to have a complete understanding of how your thoughts and beliefs can make or break your mental health. Thoughts help to form your beliefs. When you have the same thoughts repeatedly, they become beliefs. You become so used to the thoughts that they become ingrained in your subconscious, and it becomes hard to imagine that those thoughts aren't true. Accordingly, when you think negatively, you tend to have a more pessimistic outlook.

Not all thoughts are beliefs. The thoughts that come and go through your mind without repetition never become beliefs. Beliefs are a product of habitual thinking. This means that while it may be hard to break them, you can break them by overwriting those negative thoughts with positive ones, which is a practice that many therapies and techniques discussed in this book use to reduce stress, anxiety, and depression.

As you've seen with the map of reality, perception shapes our views, and it also shapes the way we think. Your thoughts build your beliefs, and your beliefs, in turn, build your sense of what's real. Some of your beliefs will empower you to seek success and find happiness, while others will make the world seem like a dark and scary place with no hope. Try to identify the parts of your belief system that cause you to have negative responses.

Your thought patterns have tremendous power to change your life. The simple act of interrupting negative thought patterns can help you begin to make changes. These changes don't happen overnight, and deeply entrenched beliefs may even take months or years to debunk completely, but, when you focus on the thought patterns you want to instill, you start to question the "truths" you blindly believed.

There will be some beliefs you'll want to keep, and those are ones you can build upon and use to your advantage throughout this process. There's no need to get rid of any belief that's constructive because such beliefs are the ones that help you grow. However, be honest about the beliefs that are hurting you. Many people try to rationalize certain beliefs that they feel psychologically unready to call into question. Open your mind and contemplate, "Is this belief hurting me in covert and manipulative ways?" If you struggle even to pose that question about a particular belief, that belief may be a harmful one.

The way you think isn't something that's out of

your control. According to the Massachusetts Institute of Technology (MIT), 45 percent of your daily choices are habitual, meaning they're a product of your subconscious thought patterns and beliefs. You choose what stimuli you feed to your subconscious. When worries or hopelessness begin to fill your head, try saying to yourself, "The world is a place full of opportunity and good things." While it won't feel like saying this is doing anything at first, rewriting your internal monologue can be a powerful first step toward growth.

When you understand how thoughts and core beliefs shape your behaviors, it becomes easier to create a path for growth. You learn that you're in charge of your beliefs, and your thoughts can only have as much control over you as you give them. You may feel helpless against your negative thoughts, but learning to overcome these harmful thoughts and release the power they have over you is the only way to become a happier person. The more you try to avoid the things that make you anxious, stressed, or depressed, the more anxious, stressed, and depressed you'll become.

Cognitive Distortions

While your brain does its best to give you helpful information and create an accurate perception of reality, sometimes it gets a little lost trying to translate what it observes into a sensible perception. Your brain loves to make connections, and sometimes, it will make connections that are overly simplified and don't show the nuance in a situation. This is called a cognitive distortion.

Simple speaking, cognitive distortions are falsehoods that your brain persuades you into believing are true. Cognitive distortions can take a variety of forms, but one common example is polarized thinking. When you think in polarities, you see things as wrong or right, good or bad, or win or lose. After you fail at one task, you may start to think, "I'll fail every task because I can't do anything right." This perception isn't an accurate one, but you become convinced it's true because your brain has pinpointed what it thinks is a pattern.

The problem with cognitive distortions is that they're often shrouded in negativity. They make you expect the worse, and they convince you that you cannot do certain things or that other things are unsafe. Cognitive distortions change your perspective, and they can quickly become harmful to your overall well-being. If you believe false messages, it's hard to make peace with your situation or feel secure. When you feel insecure, your mental health declines, and your doubts start to make it harder to function normally. Anxiety may take hold, and you may feel more stressed as you try to complete tasks. The hardship of your situation may then lead to depression.

Cognitive distortions can also cause you to act in ways that worsen your mental state. For example, someone with an eating disorder may tell themselves, "Not eating helps me," when they lose a couple of pounds. They keep going with harmful behaviors because a faulty pattern was established of believing that an action is "good," even though the behavior, for obvious reasons, is the opposite of helpful.

Likewise, someone with anxiety may say, "Avoiding this task will make me feel calmer," when procrastination only heaps on the pressure and stress of the situation. Delaying the task may have given them a sense of relief before, so they keep doing it. It continues to impair them, but cognitive distortion causes them to keep repeating the same harmful behavior. Cognitive distortions fool you into thinking certain actions are good for you or that they aren't as harmful as they are. Someone may engage in risky behavior and think, "This won't hurt me because it didn't harm me before," when that's not accurate information. People often use these distortions to justify harmful, habitual behaviors that give temporary relief to mental distress, but this causes more problems in the long run.

Negative Thoughts

Negative thoughts can play an influential role in how your brain works because your thoughts help create your map of reality and form your cognitive distortions. It's much easier to give in to negative thoughts than positive ones. People often expect the worst because they're afraid that having hope will lead to disappointment. Negative thoughts are also fueled by the internalization of negative comments that others have made about you in the past. For instance, if your mother tells you that you're ugly, you may start to think you're unattractive until it ultimately becomes a core belief.

Research has shown how much healthier and happier people are when they think positively because the brain responds to the input we give it.

So, you can change your outlook by thinking with more positivity. When you think negatively, you're feeding your brain with information it can use against you; therefore, give it information that will help you instead!

The Role of Trauma

Trauma is a significant part of human life, and it can be one of the largest contributors to adverse mental health outcomes, including increased depression, anxiety, and stress. According to the National Council for Behavioral Health, 70 percent of adults in the United States have experienced at least one traumatic event, which means that 223.4 million people in the United States alone have had trauma. Moreover, among people who seek treatment for mental health issues, 90 percent have gone through trauma. Consequently, if you have trauma, it contributes to some of the issues you may be experiencing.

Trauma is the result of events that cause deep

worry or distress. Traumatic experiences are often those that either threaten a person's life or the life or well-being of those they love.

You can have both physical and emotional trauma. Physical trauma can be a response to accidents, injuries, or other physical events. Physical trauma often can trigger emotional trauma, and the scars from emotional trauma often linger longer than those of physical trauma. Trauma can result from physical, verbal, emotional, or sexual abuse, and children who live in violent environments are at an increased risk for trauma. Some people don't realize they have trauma. They might say, "Oh, well, what I went through wasn't that bad compared to other people." However, trauma doesn't mean you were tortured or injured in unthinkable ways. The death of people you love or contracting a serious disease can also cause trauma. Anything can be traumatic if it makes you feel unsafe, so don't downplay those feelings—accept how you feel, even if you don't think it's "that bad."

When you have trauma that you haven't addressed, you're bound to have increased mental challenges. Trauma alone doesn't lead to mental illness, but it's a major contributing factor, and it drives you to rely on unhealthy coping mechanisms that do you more harm than good.

Trauma changes the way you think, which can impact your decision-making processes and your unconscious thoughts. Trauma makes your brain feel unsafe, and when your brain feels unsafe, it focuses on protecting you from future pain, because that pain could threaten your survival. Even in circumstances that don't usually cause anxiety, you may start to feel threatened, even if you can't logically explain why. When you go through trauma, your brain has a stress response, and that stress response reacts to the trauma by changing your future behaviors in an attempt to protect you.

The stress response involves areas of the brain, including the prefrontal cortex, hippocampus, and amygdala. These areas experience lingering changes when they undergo the intense pressure of trauma. As a result, the way your brain processes information shifts when you experience trauma. Your amygdala becomes more active. This part of your brain is responsible for your flight-or-fight reactions and, when it's overactive, it can make you feel as though you're in danger in non-dangerous situations. It stays on guard because it wants to prevent any potential threats from sneaking up on you.

When your amygdala becomes more active, you may be more prone to feeling stressed, and the hippocampus—the part of your brain that handles short-term memories—may become less active. As a result, you may struggle to differentiate between things that happened to you in the past and things that are presently happening.

Finally, the pre-cortex may shrink, and when it does, you have trouble dealing with your emotions and regulating your thoughts. Many of these changes can be found in people who have post-traumatic stress disorder (PTSD), but anyone with trauma can experience them to a lesser degree.

For obvious reasons, trauma makes it hard for you to be mentally healthy, but it also makes it hard for you to be physically healthy. When your physical health declines, this creates additional causes of anxiety, stress, and depression. Thus, not only can your mental health make your physical health worse, but your physical health can make your mental health worse. The Canadian Mental Health Association reports that people with depression are three times as likely to have chronic pain than people without depression. People who have chronic pain are two times as likely to have anxiety or a mood disorder. Mental and physical health are often dependent on one another, which is why the correlations between the two are so important.

According to statistics, you are more likely to experience health issues such as chronic obstructive pulmonary disease (COPD), heart disease, high blood pressure, cancer, and diabetes when you have trauma. These conditions can all reduce your life's quality or longevity, which can then create even more mental unrest. That psychological turbulence can lead to your physical conditions worsening. You can see how these situations can quickly become bleak for those experiencing them. However, by addressing your trauma, you can reduce the potency of some of these issues.

Trauma, unfortunately, is a normal part of life. For many people, it's challenging to manage, but it's nothing to be ashamed of. Using the strategies in this book, you can learn to become conscious of your trauma and take away the power it has to control your life. Simple techniques like listening to music, establishing a healthy diet and exercise routine, practicing meditation, and admitting you have trauma are just some of the most basic techniques you can use to recover.

Recovery from trauma is painful, but it's one of the most important things you can do for your health because working through trauma allows you to heal your brain and teach it new patterns.

Get Professional Help

Before you do anything, you should seek professional help. Seeing a doctor or a mental health professional can help ensure that you have a support system in place to help you improve yourself.

While this book's techniques can help you improve your levels of stress, anxiety, and depression, some people will still need professional support to help push them toward their goals. Additionally, for some people, these issues may be related to their brain chemistry, which may require medication. To have a satisfactory recovery experience, you must take a holistic approach that ensures you achieve long-lasting results and can learn coping skills that will shape the rest of your life.

Recap

Your brain is complex, and it is programmed to keep you safe and make sense of a confusing world. It uses patterns to establish norms, and those norms become the backbone of your behaviors. Your thoughts build into beliefs, and your beliefs create your worldview. Your worldview becomes your map of reality; this map is not always accurate because it's based on your brain's biases and distortions. Your brain loves finding patterns, and sometimes it finds connections that only exist in your head.

When your reality is negative and drives you

towards destructive behaviors, you need to question these beliefs and reframe your reality map. It is essential to focus on positive thoughts and vanquish negativity to create better mental health.

Further, you must learn to face the trauma you have endured because trauma changes the activity levels in the important centers of your brain. Your brain is wired to keep you safe, so trying to resist the pattern-seeking nature of your mind is fruitless; instead, you should use the way your brain works to your advantage and feed it with positive stimuli so that you have better mental health.

Finally, I urge you to seek professional help for outstanding issues as part of a holistic approach to curing your mental distress